A Simple Weight Loss Plan That Can Work for You:

How to Lose Weight Quickly in an
Atmosphere of Love
(Lose 77 Pounds Forever)

ISBN-13: 978-1974328543
ISBN-10: 1974328546

Table of Contents

Book Description

This book was written for those who almost lost hope of losing weight. For those who tried various diets but still gained weight. For those who tried to get rid of belly fat with the help of intensive training, but failed. Don't give up your dream to become slim and good-looking. Make one more attempt and read this book and you will understand that it is possible to lose 77 lbs without exhausting diets and workouts in the gym. It is based on a true life story of a man who succeeded in his last attempt to lose weight and stayed slim and athletic afterwards.

Stereotypes about everyday meals and traditional views on leisure activities result in adding weight. Step by step you will learn how to choose healthy products and regularly eat nourishing dishes that will never give you a chance to feel hunger. You will also learn how the simplest physical exercises can do miracles with your figure. The detailed and effective plan of dieting, which you can easily put into practice, will certainly help you slim down.

Besides, this book is about the atmosphere of love in which it is so easy to lose weight and reach unbelievable results. All we need for the final victory is love and sincere support of our relatives and friends. So, if you want to see your spouse slim and good-looking, this book is for you.

Last Attempt

He was 42 and had always been overweight since his childhood. Even as a kid, when his life was filled with lots of activities and sports games, he looked built more like a barrel than an average boy. And nothing had changed. Office, sofa and TV. Every single day of his life followed the same pattern. Do minimal movement and eat lots of food at one go.

The aspiring journalist, a loving husband, and a father of two beautiful children found himself caught in the vicious circle that he seemed unable to get out of. He kept gaining weight and finally reached the record 276 lbs (125 kg) and 41 inches (105 cm) in waist. Besides, he suffered from high blood pressure, dyspnea and joint pain.

He did try to lose weight a couple of times, but his attempts that seemed successful at first turned out to be a complete disaster in the very end as he put on weight again. After everything, he decided to make one more attempt. The last one. It was supposed to be a real breakthrough. Something which could help him become as slim, healthy and happy as never before.

It didn't take much to realize his dream. Seven months of hard ruthless work. Seven months that changed his attitude towards food, sports and leisure activities. From December, 2015 till June, 2016, he managed to lose 66 lbs. Instead of a corpulent figure, he got a slim and muscular body. Besides, he felt joy, satisfaction, and incredible lightness.

It is all about my husband, and I have been with him all this time. I've made up my mind to write about it. His journey to a new body was a real challenge for him but he did succeed in it.

Losing weight and not gaining it again is possible, even if you don't have:

- Lots of money to spend on food;
- The opportunity to go to healthy food restaurants;
- Sneakers for running;
- The opportunity to work out in a sports gym;
- Electronic weights for everyday weighing.

We had nothing from the list. Unfortunately, the mortgage loan for buying a one-bedroom apartment, which cost 50 000 $ with an annual 17% bank interest, came as a real burden on the family budget. So we started our work with healthy food and the simplest physical exercises.

They say there are no alcoholics who gave up drinking. And there are no overweight people who slimmed down. It's a lie. In seven months you can become the person who will never put on weight again. My husband managed to become that person.

Differences That Brought Us Closer

I have always been slim, even thin. I'm 5'8" and at the age of 36 my weight was 121 lbs (55 kg). Since my childhood I've always been told how thin I am and that I look like a lamp post, but I take this kind of jokes as a compliment, as it is so pleasant to have a slim, model-type figure. No matter how much I eat I never seem to be able to gain weight. I only added 33 lbs (15 kg) when I was expecting a baby, which I lost one year after the birth of my son.

Unlike me, my husband has always been prone to adding weight. Our marriage made our body differences grow bigger. Though we are of the same height, we ate the same food, consumed almost the same number of daily calories, I remained slim but my husband kept gaining weight. I used to bake cakes and buns, fry donuts and French fries for him. Day by day, all that yummy stuff caused a ruinous effect on his body. The truth is, I really like plump people as they seem to be very kind and gentle, but my husband didn't want to keep being overweight.

Having realized my husband's true desire to lose weight, I tried to encourage him though I went for the wrong tactic. There were jokes or direct requests that he should go on a diet. Or even worse, I would compare him with a popular and slim TV personality. No wonder, all that caused his resistance and there was no progress in the dieting results. Everything changed when I changed myself, and the atmosphere about our home.

I made up my mind to love and accept my husband the way he was - with his excessive weight, his unsuccessful attempts to lose it, his habit to lie on the sofa when I needed his hand with household chores or while taking care of our little son. I decided to keep respecting him even though he sometimes made wrong decisions, wasted our money or spent time boozing with friends. It was his life and he was responsible for it. I might not like what he did but he was a good man. And I did love him.

One evening I was preparing to go for a walk with my son while my husband was watching some endless TV series. I told him, "Have a rest. You must be tired after the working day." I closed the door even though I wanted so much for him to go for a walk with us! But he chose TV, again. Still, I decided to keep thinking positively as all I wanted was to be happy. I went out, feeling calm and cheerful at the thought that I had a beautiful son with whom I was going to spend some great time together.

When I came home I felt at once that something big was coming. And my husband suggested that maybe I should count his calories. Of course, I agreed!

Daily Calories

Actually, calories are not as important as we think they are. We ate the same amount of food, but my husband added pounds and I didn't. Though at the initial stage of losing weight, counting calories you consume can help you stay disciplined and careful while choosing what to put on your plate. We counted calories for a few weeks but very quickly understood how much we had to eat to feel sated.

Nutritionists say that people who are prone to adding weight shouldn't consume more than 2200 calories per day. My husband decided to consume 1600 calories per day. We didn't risk going for the smaller number of calories. Doctors argue that our bodies perceive a daily intake of 1200 calories as hunger. As a result, everything we eat is transformed into fat.

What can you eat or drink to get these 1600 calories? Three Snickers Super bars and as-many-as-you-want cups of tea with no sugar. But still, you will feel hungry. Instead, you can have a nice serving of porridge with salad and a small piece of meat or fish a few times a day. We opted for the latter, which seemed to be more nourishing. The idea was to eat quite a lot but it had to be a low-caloric diet. Besides, it had to supply the body with substantial quantity of vitamins and micro-elements to provide a perfect balance of proteins, fats and carbs. Proteins are the building blocks of our body, while fats and carbs give us energy.

We followed the advice given by fitness instructors who are convinced that efficient fat burning is possible when energy needs of our body are covered by 40-50% of proteins, 30-40% of carbs, and 10-20% of fats.

Daily count of calories, proteins, carbs and fats was my responsibility and it turned out to be quite a tedious task. Thus, I chose to use the mobile app that made my life much simpler. It is provided by Google Play or Apple Store and can be downloaded for free.

During the first days of dieting we realized that everyday consumption of fats exceeded all possible levels though we thought that we ate a bit of them only. Fat was lurking in beefsteaks, sausages, cheese, cream, butter, margarine, mayonnaise and various sauces.

We also consumed too many carbs; we got them from sandwiches, cakes and cookies, chocolate and sweets, Cola and juice. All these are fast carbs, which are easily digested by our body and boost the level of sugar in the blood. When it decreases, you feel hunger in no time. If you start fighting it, you only gain extra weight.

What we did lack was protein. It is an extremely important nutrient that helps form and restore muscles. And my husband wanted to have so much. Besides, protein is the safest bet from the point of view of gaining weight as its digestion takes as much energy as it brings to our body.

So my husband tried to eat lots of rich-in-protein products during the first three months of dieting. Those were: meat, fish, eggs, yogurts and cottage cheese, beans, peas, lentils and nuts.

Here is the list of typical dishes my husband had while dieting:

Breakfast
Pearl barley porridge 3.5 oz /100 gr (110 cal)
Salad with fresh lettuce and a few drops of oil 7 oz /200 gr (100 cal)
Boiled chicken breast 3.5 oz /100 gr (140 cal)

Snack 1
Sugar-free coffee (2 cal)
Bitter chocolate 1/3 oz /10 gr (55 cal)

Lunch
Pearl barley porridge 1.7 oz / 50 gr (55 cal)
Boiled chicken breast 3.5 oz / 100 gr (140 cal)
Tinned beans 5.3 oz / 150 gr (140 cal)
Whole wheat bread 1 oz / 30 gr (72 cal)
2 apples 10.5 oz / 300 gr (150 cal)

Snack 2
Sugar-free tea (0 cal)
Fat-free cottage cheese 2.5 oz / 70 gr (50 cal)
Strawberry jam 1tablespoon / 18 gr (50 cal)
Walnuts ¼ oz / 7 gr (45 cal)

Dinner
Roasted mackerel 7 oz / 200 gr (300 cal)
Boiled broccoli 3.55 oz / 100 gr (30 cal)
2 peppers (40 cal)

Snack 3
Fat-free yogurt 8 oz /170 gr (120 cal)

The total number of calories equaled 1600 calories.

Fat, Which Doesn't Kill But Heals

"Do you want to get cancer?
Fry in oil.
Do you want to die young?
Then use butter."

Elena Malysheva,
Professor, PhD and a popular TV presenter

Fat is of extremely high calorie. 1 gram of it coming into our body with food gives us 9 calories, while 1 gram of protein or 1 gram of carbs gives us only 4 calories. If you are trying to lose weight, you are to consume as little fat as possible. And that's what we did.

We tried to add less oil to salads, gave up fried food and buying cookies that contain margarine. We said "no" to fat meat, sausages, cheese and even pizza. We kissed good-bye to eating sandwiches and hamburgers. This food contains too much fat rich in cholesterol. It causes the development of atherosclerotic plagues that keep growing and blocking our blood vessels. Unfortunately, atherosclerosis leads to the development of strokes and heart attacks.

We did want fats not to kill us but to strengthen our health. Such fats exist; they contain unsaturated Omega 3 and Omega 6 fatty acids. These acids help keep the normal level of cholesterol, which prevents developing atherosclerosis. The most available source of unsaturated fatty acids is fish and linseed oil.

Doctors strongly recommend linseed oil as it is characterized by the perfect balance of Omega 3 and Omega 6 fatty acids. 1-2 tablespoonfuls of linseed oil completely satisfy the daily need of a human body for unsaturated fatty acids. We started taking 1 tablespoonful of linseed oil (7 gr) with meals on a daily basis (63 cal). It doesn't work well as a salad dressing though it is bitter in taste. To make salads we used refined olive or sunflower oil.

Doctors advise to eat fish rich in Omega 3 fatty acids at least two times a week. Salmon and trout are very expensive in our country. We couldn't afford to buy such fish even one time a month. We chose a cheaper option - herring and mackerel. Quite often we had it cooked in oven with herbs and pepper. Also, we began eating tinned sardine, saury and tuna.

Sometimes we took linseed oil at intervals. Besides, we couldn't buy fish on a regular basis. When it happened, we took fish oil in capsules that we ordered at iHerb.com, the biggest internet site selling vitamins, nutritional supplements and natural health products. 2 capsules containing 2 grams of fish oil completely cover the daily need of a human body for vitamin D and Omega 3 fatty acids.

Instead of sweets with our tea and coffee, we began eating nuts, sunflower and pumpkin seeds, which are rich in unsaturated fatty acids and vitamins and contain no cholesterol.

Right now, we try to avoid fried meals because at high temperatures oil turns into transformed fat with devastating effect on our blood vessels and causing atherosclerosis. What's more important, when oil gets heated poly-aromatic hydrocarbons are formed, which can lead to cancer. The best option is not to fry but roast. When oil is diluted with water, the boiling temperature gets lower. So, changes in oil won't be as radical as during the frying process.

Besides, we gave up eating margarine. As it turned out, it is actually transformed fat and an extremely harmful product. It is made of vegetable oil, but unlike it, margarine is solid. Oil undergoes the process of hydrogenation; it turns into solid because unsaturated fatty acids are transformed into saturated ones. Margarine is No.1 enemy of our blood vessels. If you happen to have it in your fridge, just throw it into your garbage bin.

There is too much transformed fat in cookies and cakes, sweets and chocolate bars, and also in French fries. Fat-containing products can provoke weight gain while natural products usually don't have such effect.

Proper Carbs

Carbs help us stay active all day long. Our family used to get them from harmful products. Those were white bread, sweets, pasta, soda. We decided to have them substituted with vegetables and fruit. They are rich in carbohydrates, get digested for quite a long time and help us feel sated.

Vegetables and fruit are rich in cellulose that helps clean our intestine. Cellulose itself is almost calories-free, but in our stomach it gets swollen and gives us the feeling of being sated. Thus, we don't get hungry for a while.

One more source of cellulose is bran. We bought oat, wheat, rye bran and added it almost to every dish: pancakes, porridge, and even muffins.

We call bran pieces of grain husk separated from flour after milling. Bran is usually used to feed animals. So they eat the most useful part of the grain!

For centuries our ancestors used to eat dark bread made of wholegrain wheat. People baked bread with white flour on very special occasions. White bread is really very tasty, soft and tender, but it lacks vitamins and micro-elements.

To make refined flour that can be kept for a long time they separate it both from bran and nucleus rich in vitamin E and micro-elements. They also get rid of aleurone, protein stored as granules in the cells of plant seeds. What is left in refined wheat after processing? Actually, nothing except useless calories.

On learning that, we began to use wholegrain flour in cooking and buy wholegrain bread in the supermarket. It might not be super tasty, but it is super useful!

We got used to eating lots of vegetables and fruit, but sometimes we just couldn't afford to buy them because of the huge mortgage loan we had to pay back. It made us look for the alternative ways and we went for cereals.

The staples of our diet became various kinds of porridge made of oatmeal, buckwheat, rice, rye, pearl barley and wheat. Cooking porridge takes quite a long period of time, that's why we chose to leave cereals covered in water overnight, and in the morning we boiled them in a matter of 15-20 minutes. These cereals contain complex carbohydrates. You are guaranteed to feel sated after such meals for quite a long time as they are slowly digested by our body filling it with energy.

One more important aspect of dieting is unrefined cereals. They are rich in proteins, carbs, fats, cellulose, vitamins B1 and E, mineral elements (iron, phosphorus). Quite surprisingly, cereals contain the optimal balance of them, which makes them the best choice for everybody.

If you so much like rice, you can eat it on a daily basis, though you should keep in mind that it should be brown (unpolished). If it is polished it loses its nucleus, which makes it white, quick to boil and pleasant in taste. So it has no useful elements left, nor bran or nucleus. If you keep it in water, it will never grow. Such kind of rice is "dead". Brown (unpolished) rice is the opposite of it; it is the kind of live food we need for healthy life.

Protein Trap

"Do you really think that the omnivores lion possesses extraordinary muscles? The truth is, the herbivores, such as the horse and the deer, have no worse muscles. The lion's advantage is its unexpected lightning-like dash as it can't chase a prey for a long time. The lion knows it has no chances of catching its prey if it runs for long."

Hiromi Shinja,
one of the world's leading gastroenterologists

At the initial stage of our dieting, we ate quite a lot of meat dishes and eggs. My husband has always been an avid lover of meat. It caused no difficulties for him to give up eating sweets and fatty products but he had to substitute them with something as his appetite never disappeared. So, he decided to go in for chicken breasts and eggs as the most available source of protein needed for growing muscles. Porridge, vegetables and fruit were also part of his diet but meat always prevailed.

Having read lots of fitness instructors' advice on the topic, my husband persisted on convincing me that he had to get 1.2-1.5 gr of protein per 1 kg of his weight a day. It resulted in consumption of 4.2-5.2 oz (120-150 gr) of protein that he got from meat and dairy products as his desired weight was 220 lbs (100 kg) at the time. We had meat courses for breakfast, lunch and dinner.

The diet, which consisted of 40-50% protein calories, 30-40% carb calories and 10-20% fat calories, really helped achieve unbelievable results. We realized it when my husband first weighed while visiting my sister. During the first month of dieting, he lost 15.5 lbs (7 kg). The next two months helped him shed 28.5 lbs (13 kg).

I was aware that further protein diet could cause problems in kidney functioning, poisoning the body with protein processing products and even cancer. I tried my best to convince my husband that too much protein could be harmful, but he wouldn't listen.

I chose to stop talking to him on the topic. I was just hoping for some kind of miracle. Quite soon he happened to read the book "Enzyme Factor", written by one the best modern Japanese gastroenterologists and surgeons, Hiromi Shinya. In the book, he proves the falsity of the men's stereotype that you can't become muscular with eating no meat.

His book suggests that big quantities of animal origin protein speed up our body development, which is probably the main reason of acceleration. But there is danger hiding here as meat speeds up both development and ageing processes.

Another book, which helped change my husband's views on protein was "Finding Ultra: Rejecting Middle Age, Becoming One of the World's Fittest Men, and Discovering Myself" by Rich Roll. The former alcoholic who used to suffer from obesity succeeded in becoming one of the 25 strongest men in the world. In 2010, the sportsman managed to meet the unbelievable endurance challenge, Epic 5. In one week he managed to cover 5 triathlon distances (12 mile swim in open water, 560 mile bike race, followed by a full 131 mile marathon).

He managed to do it as a vegan, which meant receiving all necessary protein from vegetable food. Besides, he consumed no more than 1 gr of it per 1 kg of weight a day. It completely changed my husband's point of view about the impossibility of being an achiever in sports without meat protein consumption. It made us change our approach and now only 12-15% of our daily calories consist of proteins.

Proteins can be obtained from various sources, not only from animal origin products. For example, 9 indispensable amino acids, which are contained in proteins, can be received from wheat, nuts, seeds, vegetables and beans. Indispensable amino acids can be found in various kinds of beans, almonds, lentils, spinach and broccoli. All these products became a part of our diet. We began consuming less meat but the process of losing weight never stopped.

Giving Up Milk

While dieting, my husband consumed lots of milk protein coming from milk, yogurt, cheese and curd. Trying to reduce the quantities of protein, we gradually gave up eating dairy products. It was no easy decision to make. Dairy products used to be the staples since our childhood and it was almost impossible to imagine our life without them. We were convinced it would result in serious problems with our teeth as they would lack calcium.

It's a well-known fact that milk contains a unique combination of proteins, fats, carbohydrates, calcium and vitamin D. But recent studies make us change our attitude about milk. As it turns out, milk might become a cause of an untimely death.

Besides, a few years ago, the alliance of doctors of Harvard medical school excluded milk from the list of products useful to our health.

The most harmful for a human body is beef fat found in dairy products. Its so-called solid fat litters our organism with cholesterol and causes atherosclerotic plaques in the blood vessels. To stay healthy one can buy non-fat milk, but still that doesn't make it the absolutely safe product.

Modern milk production is part of a huge manufacturing process; cows can be milked up to 300 days a year while the usual period of lactation for a cow is 180 days a year only. How can this fact be explained? Livestock is fed with specially-developed fodder containing estrone sulfate hormone, which stimulates lactation. According to the latest research, its level is 33% higher in farm than free-range livestock. Estrone sulfate hormone can be the cause of prostate and testicles cancer. It should be mentioned also that calves, if fed with milk bought at the supermarket, die on the fourth or fifth day of their lives.

It was my son, David who made me pay particular attention to the use of milk. While breastfeeding him, I ate lots of dairy products and he got ill quite often. Since his birth he suffered from lactase insufficiency; his organism lacked lactase enzyme that is crucial in processing the milk sugar called lactose. As it turned out, every fourth person in the world cannot digest milk because of lactase insufficiency.

The older we get the less lactase we get produced in our body. Elderly people can easily develop diarrhea as a consequence of drinking one glass of milk. As for dairy products, they are better digested as they contain less lactase. So people who can't drink milk can still consume yogurts and various cheeses.

One more curious fact is that milk is on the list of 9 products that cause allergic reactions. One of the most widespread allergic reactions among children is the one caused by cow milk protein.

According to the latest researches, people break bones more often in the countries with the highest milk consumption. The other proved fact is that in such countries bigger numbers of people suffer from diabetes. So, is it worthwhile for adults to drink milk?

In the wildlife, there are no animals feeding on milk all their life. They drink only their mother's milk and only for a certain period of time. For example, elk's foul starts feeding on grass soon after its birth. Grass contains sufficient quantity of calcium to help the bones grow.

While breastfeeding my son I stopped eating all dairy products except butter for 9 months, as I followed our pediatrician's advice which was aimed at preventing rash and diarrhea. I was afraid that I was going to get a huge cavity in each of my teeth because of the lack of calcium. I substituted dairy products with broccoli, tinned sardine and saury, added poppy and sesame seeds to dishes, and also took calcium supplements. When I got an appointment with my dentist, he assured me that all my teeth were absolutely healthy.

The doctors reveal surprising calcium sources you can add to your diet if you choose to live without milk. Calcium-rich foods: kale, oranges, sardines, soy milk, oatmeal, sesame seeds, Swiss cheese, soybeans, almonds, salmon, white beans, yogurt, dried figs, turnip greens, arugula, broccoli, tofu, sunflower seeds.

Cow milk can also be substituted with coconut or rice milk. In this case your body will get useful vegetable fat instead of harmful beef fat.

Getting Rid of the Old Illness

For many years my husband suffered from a disease, which didn't let him go anywhere without socks. It was psoriasis. And he had big red spots on both feet he would carefully hide from people. Quite surprisingly, they disappeared when my husband radically changed his diet.

Modern scientists are still uncertain about the reasons people develop psoriasis, though there are a few popular diets recommending to stop eating citrus fruits, chocolate, eggs, honey, whole milk and products containing red pigment (tomatoes, strawberries, etc.) All these products, except milk, are still a part of my husband's diet. It makes me think that giving up milk, which he used to drink a couple of glasses every day, was the main reason for his recovery.

There was also a 1$ Chinese-make ointment that helped speed up his recovery. We read buyers' reviews and ordered it at Chinese online shopping website AliExpress.com. After a one-week use, all the red spots were gone and the disease never came back.

Rucksack Full of Food to Lose Weight

"Just think about it: we are fed every 2-3 hours, 7-8 times a day when we are born. And this is right... In that case, why do we stop eating regularly when we get to our working place? Why do we get convinced that our main priority is work and not our body?"

Margarita Koroleva,
a nutritionist who runs a clinic of aesthetic medicine

One of the secrets of successful weight loss was my husband's habit to take short intervals between meals to prevent his body from getting the feeling of hunger. Our body must know it is loved and regularly fed. If so it won't start storing fat for the fear it will have to diet next day.

If we eat only few times a day it means that we eat a lot. In fact, we overeat 1 or 2 times a day, which is a real challenge for a digesting system and a cause of obesity.

My husband succeeded in keeping the magic feeling of being sated, as he always takes a rucksack full of food to his work. I sometimes joke that all his colleagues would be wishing they could go on a diet like him even when the various tasty dishes he eats just makes him lose weight.

We go neither to fast food places nor to any other restaurants. That is why, taking some food along is a reliable and quite affordable way to stay sated all day.

When my husband started a dieting regime he followed the rule of 5-6 meals per day. And now it has become "the golden standard" for every day: breakfast, snack 1, lunch, snack 2, dinner, and sometimes snack 3. Here are the details:

Breakfast at 7.30 am before leaving home for work. It usually consists of wholegrain wheat porridge with a piece of boiled or roasted meat (sometimes it is substituted with corn, lentils or beans). After that, he works in the office till 5.30 pm. A year ago, during his lunch time, he used to go to McDonald's restaurant. Other times, he ate a ham sandwich taken from home. I realized how often he went to fast food restaurants when I opened his desk drawer and found a huge heap of paper bags that came from French fries and hamburgers.

After such dinners, my husband would eat as a horse in the evening as he felt very hungry and exhausted. 5-hour intervals between meals are no good for people trying to get rid of some extra pounds. Our body feels stress and won't give away fat stores, which slows down the process of losing weight.

When snacks came into my husband's life, the task of slimming down became so easy! At 9 am, my husband takes a cup of sugar-free coffee and a small piece of dark chocolate with candied oranges (1/3 oz / 10 gr), eats 2 or 3 dried dates or a few raisins, and a bit of sunflower seeds.

He eats lunch at 12.30 pm. It is usually brought from home and consists of wholegrain porridge, salad, 1 boiled egg (fish, meat, beans). He eats 2 apples for the dessert on a regular basis. In the summertime, he can go for a few pieces of melon or water melon, or a handful of berries (bilberries, strawberries, grapes).

3.30 pm is the time of snack 2. It usually consists of sugar-free tea and 2 crispbreads with peanut butter, though they can be substituted with a banana, an apple or a piece of cheese.

Traditionally, we have dinner at 6.30 pm. We usually have vegetable soup with a piece of bread, baked pumpkin and tinned beans.

Following this diet my husband tried to reduce his servings. Once he said that he felt sated after eating only half of what he had on the plate, he stopped overeating and it was so unusual!

Our family do get snacks before going to bed. We enjoy sitting at the table and talking about things happening in our lives. That is why, at 8-9 pm we can have a cup of tea with some dietary biscuits or eat a few big pieces of water melon. And my husband has no pangs of remorse doing it! I also stopped worrying about the bad effects of late snacks as after 3 months of dieting he started going in for sports.

Life Full of Movement

"If you want to run, run in your smart shoes."

Radislav Gandapas,
a business coach and a specialist in leadership

My husband's previous attempts to lose weight failed because they were only about a rigid diet regime. His life lacked movement, and as a consequence of that he would always gain weight again. This time, our choice was to move a lot every day. I used to have walks with my son alone, but now my husband started sharing our company.

When we had no money to buy gas for the car, we never got upset. Our financial difficulties are a temporary thing, we knew it. That is why we appreciated our subway trips as they gave us a chance for additional exercising.

The breaking point for my husband was his decision to walk 1.8 miles (3 km) in 30 minutes every day. No matter what the weather was like, what mood he was in, or what his colleagues thought about it, he firmly resolved to become the black sheep of the family. And unlike his colleagues who stay in, he goes out for a walk during his lunch time.

If you repeat a certain action 13 times, it becomes your habit. And if you get used to something, it feels bad to change the set order - writes Erik Bertrand Larssen in his bestseller "No Mercy. Be Your Best With Mental Training". This piece of advice helped lots of businessmen and sportsmen to reach their goals in quite challenging conditions. My husband followed it too.

He didn't miss a single workout session. He also sets reminders on his phone to make it easier for him to stand up and go for a walk after lunch. We live in a metropolis that lacks parks and green zones. That is why, a 1.8 mile (3-km) distance for him means a walk along busy streets in the downtown. During his walks he burnt about 350 calories. During a period of 6 months he covered a distance of 223 miles (360 km) in his smart shoes, as he had no sneakers.

The other foundation of his success became the regular physical exercises he did at home 2 or 3 times a week. He began with warming up, then added push-ups on fists, squatting and exercises for his abdominal muscles. Now his evening workout session burns 500 calories and includes:

Warm-up
Squats - 20 reps per 3 sets
Push-ups on fists - 20 reps per 3 sets
Abs crunches - 20 reps per 2 sets
3-minute jogging between reps in our 162-square-feet (15-square-meter) bedroom.

When my husband ordered his first pair of Mizuno Wave Enigma 5 Running Shoes at Amazon.com, our life became even more exciting. One Saturday morning we drove to the park to go on a 3-mile (5-km) hiking tour with our 3-year-old son riding a bicycle. It was his first marathon!

One week later, walking was substituted with jogging. Covering a 3-mile (5-km) distance, my husband burnt 600 calories. One month later he ran 6 miles (10 km) and burnt a record-breaking 1450 calories. After such energy-consuming trainings he could eat whatever he wanted; an ice cream or pasta with his favorite sauce.

And he kept losing weight! During his first month of dieting he lost 15.5 lbs (7 kg). During the next two months he lost 28.5 lbs (13 kg). After 4 months of dieting and doing sports activities he lost additional 22 lbs (10 kg). All in all, he got rid of 66 lbs (30 kg).

Jogging and running are incredibly stimulating. They help burn fat, not muscle mass if you stick to certain rules. You should go jogging or running for at least 40 minutes, though 60 minutes is a much better option. Your body first burns carbohydrates for 20-30 minutes, and only after then does it start burning adipose tissue.

Also, it is important that you control your pulse. It should be aerobic, which means that your heart beats with sufficient frequency to provide oxygen delivery to all body tissues. Aerobic pulse is the most effective in fat burning.

If you don't control your heart beat rate while running, it can result in harmful effect on its functions. On the contrary, your workout with aerobic pulse becomes cardio-training that strengthens the heart and helps burn fat.

How can we calculate our pulse to keep it in the aerobic limits? Here is the formula: (220 - age) x 0.6-0.8, where 0.6 is the low level and 0.8 is the upper level of the aerobic pulse. For my 42-year-old husband, it must be 107-142 beats per minute, and he would always control it to stay in the normal range.

Water That Became Tasty

To lose weight you need to drink lots of water. Non-carbonated water. Not juice, tea or coffee, but fresh, clean and not very tasty water. Why? The truth is, everything except water is food and needs digesting. Besides, tea and coffee dehydrate our body, hindering the process of fat oxidation.

When we drink enough water, the cholesterol level decreases. The more water we drink, the better the metabolism and blood circulation we get. Fresh water contains no calories. If your drink contains sugar, which means empty calories, you usually have more of it in comparison with fresh water consumption. As a consequence, you gain weight. What's even more important, sweet drinks increase the level of glucose in the blood. And when it goes down, hunger returns.

Every time my husband tried to go on a diet he made a firm resolution. He always said he'd drink a lot of water, at least 4 pints (2 liters) a day, but every time he failed to realize his intentions. He failed to practice his theory. That may have been the reason for his unsuccessful previous attempts. He would forget to drink it in the morning, in the afternoon and in the evening. Even when we could afford to buy high-quality bottled water or it was provided free in the office, we would choose tea or coffee, though we shouldn't.

If you drink lots of non-carbonated water, it does help you to lose weight. Since you can easily confuse hunger with thirst, you should better have some water first than start chewing something. Besides, if you drink water 30-60 minutes before a meal, you won't feel hunger and will eat less.

Before morning grooming and breakfast, my husband drinks 1 cup (glass) of water (250 ml). He makes this morning water very tasty as he adds 1 tablespoonful of apple vinegar and honey to it. He really enjoys it. This water stimulates metabolism and strengthens his immune system.

Apple vinegar contains calcium, which is beneficial to the heart, along with 20 vital mineral and micro-elements, and a number of vitamins. Honey is very useful too. So, this morning fruit water is both tasty and rich in necessary elements for our body.

Though we drink a lot of fresh water every day, we didn't give up on the pleasure of getting tea or coffee. During snack 1, my husband has a cup of coffee. 30 minutes before his lunch at 12 pm he drinks 2 glasses of water. After his afternoon walk, he drinks another glass of water. During snack 2, he has a cup of tea (black, green, or fruit). Before dinner, at 6 pm, he again drinks a glass of water. If he has evening training he drinks additional 2 glasses of water. If not, he drinks 1 glass of water. All in all, that is 4 pints (2 liters) of water per day.

With such tough water consuming regime, you will have no time to eat! Though you will have to visit the toilet quite often, which is not so bad, after all it means additional physical activity and burning of calories.

Bread That Disappeared from Our Table

Changes that I noticed in my husband were fantastic. He began losing weight, smiled more often, and even cooked. It wasn't just omelette or porridge; he learnt how to bake sourdough bread without yeast, as it isn't the best option for us.

Baking yeast is the common name for the strains of yeast commonly used as a leavening agent in baking bread and bakery products, where it converts the fermentable sugars present in the dough into carbon dioxide and ethanol. It was specially developed to make the baking process shorter.

Active use of baking yeast started in the 1940s. Before that time breads were baked with hops, malt, rye and other kinds of sourdough, and its baking was like a ritual for every family. The recipe of the family sourdough was passed on from one generation to another. Besides, bread was made of quality wholegrain flour and was much more useful in comparison with the one we buy nowadays.

Why is baking yeast more common these days than sourdough? The answer is quite evident. It is much easier and less time-consuming to bake bread using yeast. On the contrary, sourdough needs lots of care and certain temperature conditions.

My husband learnt how to make sourdough by himself! In a big bowl he mixed rye wholegrain flour with water and let it ferment till the morning. Every day he mixed the thick substance adding some water and flour. He repeated the process for 5 days. The sourdough increased in volume, and small bubbles with pleasant sour-milk smell would appear. In such a way, the process of natural fermentation of rye flour in warm water took place in an open space where the air contains a certain number of lactic bacteria.

Then sourdough was mixed with wheat flour and miraculously it made the dough increase 2 times in volume. We got delicious homemade bread that tasted like the Italian ciabatta. It is very nutritious and gives lots of energy. Sourdough bread became a real culinary masterpiece for my husband. I learnt to bake it too. Such bread can be baked once in a week. A loaf of it can be kept for a few days as it never gets mold. Soon they started selling wholegrain sourdough bread at the local supermarket, and we buy it when we don't have time to bake it ourselves.

Everyday Meals: by Way of Simplicity

Having gone through all the dieting stages, we came to the conclusion that the simpler you cook the more useful food you get. It does good for your figure and helps you save up time. We even stopped making video recipes for our YouTube channel and became less active on Instagram, which is full of culinary masterpieces photos.

Right now our meals are quite simple. The staples are vegetables, fruit and porridge. We don't eat much meat and fish; they make up only 10-15% of our dishes. We love homemade wholegrain bread, seeds and dried fruit, but we don't go to the extremes. Sometimes we buy ice cream, and while visiting friends we never refuse to eat a piece of cake or a couple of sweets.

Thanks to the healthy diet, my husband keeps losing weight. During the one month I spent writing this book he got rid of additional 11 lbs (5 kg). I also managed to lose 6.6 lbs (3 kg) as I started jogging with him. Now my task is to gain some muscle mass.

The thought of how little food a human being needs came to me when I tried fasting for the first time in my life. I gave up eating for a day to get concentrated on my spiritual goals. When your stomach is empty and the right thoughts come to your mind, you begin to realize quite clearly how much money is wasted on useless things. We poison our body with unhealthy food, we buy clothes we wear a couple of times only and then just store in wardrobes. We get our heads stuffed with nonsense while watching primitive TV shows and soap operas. Maybe the time has come to get rid of all this rubbish and never amass it again?

More Than Just Support

Each of us needs help and encouragement at the crucial moments of our lives. For an overweight person who decides to lose weight, a switch for a new, healthy diet can turn out to be quite stressful. That is why, support from relatives and friends makes overcoming difficulties much easier. Love them the way they are, and they will become slim and beautiful!

Love means not only words, but also your actions. Are you ready to show your love in these ways?:

Are you ready to get up early to cook healthy breakfast for your close/dearest/beloved person and pack a lunch-box to take to the office? Are you ready to deprive yourself sleep?

Are you ready not to eat the very last apple remaining in the fridge and give it to your close/dearest/beloved person so that he/she could take it to work?

Are you ready not to say a word when a person near you is going through "a food breakdown" and eating unhealthy and harmful stuff? Are you ready not to notice this mistake and not to pay attention to it? Are you ready not to criticize mentally, but to wish him/her a victory next day?

Are you ready to do everything to help your close/dearest/beloved person find time to go in for sports? Are you ready to go for a walk with your child while he/she has a workout at home? Are you ready to go behind with your child when he/she runs his/her first 3-mile (5-km) distance? Are you ready to stay in the shadow to let him/her bask in the glory of victory?

Are you ready to fill the home atmosphere with love that can encourage your close/dearest/beloved person to change, to become better and to start with his/her own body transformation?

Then your close/dearest/beloved person will definitely succeed, and your family will become not only slim and athletic but also friendly and loving!

Overweight Body as a Good Start

On his 43rd birthday, my husband celebrated with the weight of 199 lbs (90 kg) and a waist of 36.6 inches (94 cm). This means he is no longer in the group with the risk of untimely death caused by stroke or heart attack.

Observing my husband, I came to realize that nothing is accidental in life. Everything is given to us for a good reason. Even our body is prone to adding weight. The truth is, it is a perfect instrument to work at oneself.

Don't feel sad if you don't look like a model. When overweight people start working at their body, incredible changes start taking place in their life. They become beautiful both in looks and in the inside. Their family life improves, they find good friends and a new job. They are full of joy and happiness. The whole world around changes for them as they change themselves.

Leave a Review

If you liked **A Simple Weight Loss Plan That Can Work for You**, please be kind enough to post a short review on Amazon.

Here is the link: **http://amzn.to/2fsqvud**

Thank you for your support.

9 781974 328543